AF711751

Go-To Guide for Phonological Awareness

Angela Sterling-Orth

THINKING PUBLICATIONS®

Thinking Publications • Eau Claire, Wisconsin

© 2004 by Thinking Publications

Thinking Publications grants limited rights to individual professionals to reproduce and distribute pages that indicate duplication is permissible. Pages can be used for instruction only and must include Thinking Publications' copyright notice. All rights are reserved for pages without the permission-to-reprint notice. No part of these pages can be reproduced in any form, electronic or mechanical, including photocopy, recording, or any information storage and retrieval system, without permission in writing from the publisher.

11 10 09 08 07 06 05 8 7 6 5 4 3 2

Library of Congress Cataloging-in-Publication Data

Sterling-Orth, Angela, date
Go to guide for phonological awareness / Angela Sterling-Orth.
p. cm.
Includes bibliographical references.
ISBN 1-932054-18-9 (pbk.)
1. Speech therapy for children. 2. English language—Phonology. I. Title.

RJ496.S7S737 2004
618.92'85506—dc22

2004046021

Printed in the United States of America

Cover design by Debbie Olson

THINKING PUBLICATIONS®
A Division of McKinley Companies, Inc.

424 Galloway Street • Eau Claire, WI 54703
715.832.2488 • Fax 715.832.9082
Email: custserv@ThinkingPublications.com

COMMUNICATION SOLUTIONS THAT CHANGE LIVES®

To J.H. and C.J.—

A father and son who make mommy's job easy

About the Author

Angela Sterling-Orth, MS, CCC-SLP, is an associate lecturer and clinical supervisor in the Department of Communication Disorders at the University of Wisconsin—Eau Claire. Ms. Sterling-Orth teaches undergraduate and graduate coursework related to serving children with communication disorders in the public schools. In addition, she supervises students working with preschool and school-age children with speech and language disorders, both in the university clinic and as they student-teach in the schools. Angie has co-authored *Silly Sounds Playground,* the *Working Out* series, and *Interactive BigBooks:* S *Clusters*—all with Thinking Publications.

Contents

Preface

This text was written out of a clear necessity—my own!

Back in the late '80s and early '90s, as I traveled through my undergraduate and graduate programs in communication disorders, the notion of understanding and targeting phonological awareness skills in children with speech and language disorders was not explicitly discussed. While the importance of phonological awareness was undoubtedly understood by my professors, calling too much attention to this area had fallen aside, as whole-language and more global issues of literacy had come to the forefront.

After I graduated and began working in the public schools as a speech-language pathologist, I began to have discussions with colleagues about improving children's phonological awareness skills and preventing reading failure. In the mid-'90s, as I moved from an early-childhood setting to a middle-school position, support for evaluating and teaching phonological awareness skills to children with speech and language difficulties grew stronger. Once again, professionals in reading instruction, learning disabilities, general education, and speech-language pathology were coming together to rediscover and describe the significance of phonological awareness skills in literacy development.

As I moved to the university setting and began working as an associate lecturer, I found myself overwhelmed with journal articles, assessment and intervention kits, and textbook chapters on phonological awareness development, disorders, and instruction. I was presenting my students with bits and pieces of information from dozens of resources. In an attempt to bring some organization to this information, this text was born.

I hope *Go-To Guide for Phonological Awareness* becomes a helpful tool to those who are trying to understand this material for the first time. And I hope it is equally helpful to those who are already versed in this information but are looking for a handy guide that has pulled everything together for easy access.

I wish to thank many individuals for their inspiration, support, and guidance as I created and polished this resource. Kris Retherford, my mentor since I was an undergraduate in the field, discovered my clinical handout on this topic and encouraged me to develop it further and submit it for publication. It would not have been "found" if it wasn't for her. Linda Schreiber and Nancy McKinley at

Thinking Publications, my professional guardian angels for the past 15 years, welcomed my submission and made the publication process painless. My undergraduate and graduate student clinicians at the University of Wisconsin—Eau Claire embraced the notion of working on phonological awareness with children who have speech and language disorders and were hungry for this knowledge. To all those students, this is for you! Finally, to my field reviewers—Julie Miller, Cindy Rieck, Robin S. Kanis, and Casey O'Keefe—this resource would not have been complete without their incredible contributions.

Special thanks to Vicki Lord Larson and Linda Schreiber who guided this project from the start. Thanks for the encouragement and leadership. My appreciation goes to Debbie Olson, graphic artist at Thinking Publications, for using her artistic talents to bring my project to life. Thanks also to my editors, Vicki Fields and Sarah Thurs, whose gentle suggestions and technical skills made this resource user-friendly and complete.

Introduction

Go-To Guide for Phonological Awareness is a reference tool providing a concise overview of phonological awareness. While you may choose to read this book from cover to cover, it is designed to allow you to quickly pick out just the information you need. The following provides a breakdown of the 5 areas of phonological awareness covered in this *Go-To Guide:*

Key Terms—Defines and explains the terms needed as a foundation for understanding phonological awareness

Importance—Explains how phonological awareness is related to literacy and to speech and language development

Development—Provides general guidelines for the typical development of 3 phonological awareness skills: word and syllable awareness, rhyme awareness, and phoneme awareness

Assessment—Describes the pros and cons of using informal and formal procedures to assess phonological awareness

Intervention—Presents considerations and guidelines for effectively teaching phonological awareness

In addition, there are 2 handy appendices you can photocopy and use when working with children: a screening checklist **(Appendix A)** and an inventory for identifying children's strengths and weaknesses **(Appendix B)**. Also included are 3 appendices to help you in your work: a summary of 9 formal assessment batteries **(Appendix C)**, a listing of nearly two dozen recommended resources to use when teaching phonological awareness skills **(Appendix D)**, and 6 example scripts describing how to use children's books to teach phonological awareness **(Appendix E)**.

A variety of educational professionals (e.g., reading teachers, psychologists, linguists, and special education teachers) have defined, described, researched, and prescribed methods for phonological awareness. This resource attempts to summarize and find points of consensus wherever disagreement may exist.

The following individuals (including students studying these professions) may find this text useful:

- Speech-language pathologists who work with preschool and school-age children
- Special education teachers (including learning disabilities teachers, teachers of students who have cognitive disabilities, and early childhood educators)
- General education teachers at both the preschool and school-age levels
- Reading teachers (including Title 1 and Reading Recovery teachers)
- Paraprofessionals who work with children who have speech, language, learning, and reading disorders
- Parents who have an interest in this topic and their child's education

Key Terms

The list of terms that comprise a complete understanding of phonological awareness seems unending. However, knowledge of several key terms is critical to understanding phonological awareness well enough to successfully evaluate an individual's awareness and provide remediation for this aspect of development. The terms defined and described in this section include the following:

- alphabetic principle
- decoding
- dyslexia
- graphemes
- language disorder
- learning disability
- metaphonological awareness
- morphological awareness
- onset
- phonemic awareness
- phonics
- phonological awareness
- phonological processing
- phonology
- reading disability
- rhyming
- rime
- specific language impairment
- word and syllable awareness

Phonological Awareness

Through the years, **phonological awareness** has been defined in a number of ways. The following is a sample of how various authors have explained this concept. Put together, they help form a comprehensive definition.

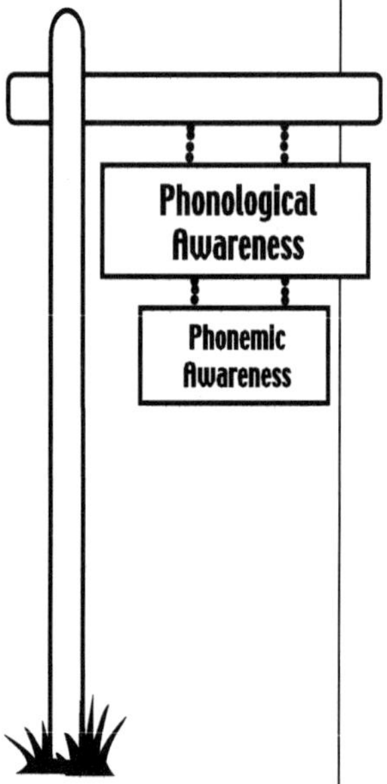

- The explicit knowledge of, awareness of, or sensitivity to the phonological structure of language; skills used to think about, compare, and manipulate sounds in words (Stanovich, 1988)
- Knowing the ways in which language (e.g., sentences and words) can be divided into smaller units (e.g., words, syllables, and sounds; Goswami & Bryant, 1990)
- Skills allowing a person to attend to the sounds of language and understand that they are distinct from the meaning, including the skills of rhyming, counting syllables, segmenting words into syllables and sounds, and recognizing onset and rime in words (Snow, Burns, & Griffin, 1998)
- A person's awareness of the sound system of language; a sensitivity that allows a person to make judgments about, or manipulate, sounds and syllables (Catts, 2000)

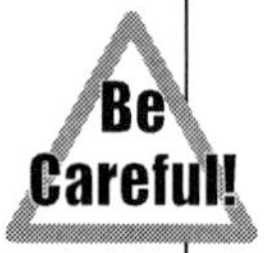

The term **phonemic awareness** is sometimes inappropriately used interchangeably with the term *phonological awareness.* Phonemic awareness is actually a subskill of phonological awareness. Because phonemic awareness occurs at the most basic (i.e., phoneme) level, it does not refer to rhyming skills or to word awareness and syllable awareness (such as in word counting, syllable segmentation, and syllable blending). Phonemic awareness specifically refers to the following:

- The understanding that words are composed of phonemes/sounds (Torgesen, 1999)
- The knowledge that phonemes have distinctive features (Torgesen, 1999)

- The awareness that words and syllables are a sequence of phonemes (Swank, 1997)
- The ability to detect, blend, segment, and manipulate sounds in words

---

Metaphonological Awareness

A less-often mentioned term in the area of phonological awareness is **metaphonological awareness.** Metaphonological awareness goes a step beyond phonological awareness in that it includes a person's skill in rhyming and in segmenting, blending, and manipulating syllables and sounds, AND in talking about these acts and then reflecting on the processes involved (Gombert, 1992). For example, a child may begin to rhyme spontaneously at age 3 or 4 and can be overheard rattling off a string of rhyming words like *"fat, cat, sat, mat"* (i.e., phonological awareness). However, that same child may not have explicit awareness of his ability to rhyme (i.e., metaphonological awareness) if he cannot respond appropriately when asked to say a word that rhymes with *dog.*

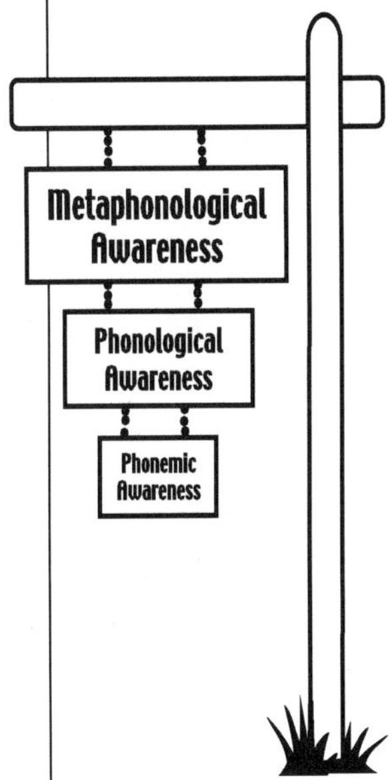

Children not only need to demonstrate phonological awareness skills, they also need to be able to talk about and explain their use of such skills. Children who do not naturally develop metaphonological awareness need instruction that models and mediates these skills (Gombert, 1992). The "Intervention" section (beginning on page 25) explains how to help children's phonological awareness skills become "meta."

For the purposes of this resource, the term *phonological awareness,* rather than *metaphonological awareness,* is used in order to remain consistent with the terminology that appears in most research and commercially available resources on this subject. Thus, the explicit knowledge that Gombert (1992) describes as metaphonological awareness is being assumed in the use of the term *phonological awareness* in this guide.

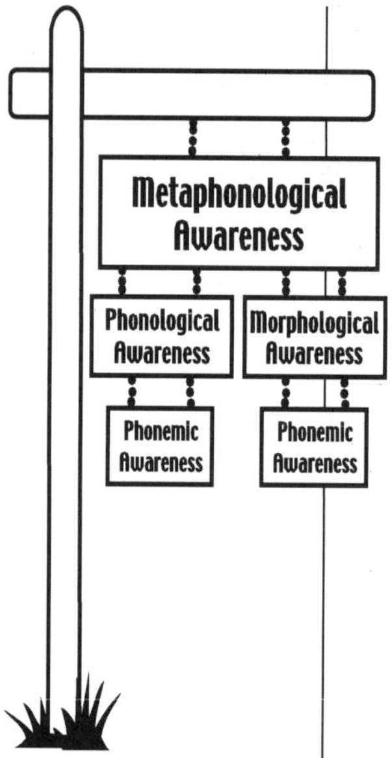

Morphological Awareness

Morphological awareness—explicit knowledge of the internal structure of words (Windsor & Hwang, 1999)—emerges as a child develops sufficient phonemic awareness. Morphological awareness includes phonemic awareness skills and applies these skills to the relationships between root words and their derivations (Masterson & Crede, 1999). This results in the recognition that phoneme changes can create a change in meaning (see Table 1).

Table 1 **Phonemic vs. Morphological Awareness**

	Phonemic Awareness	Morphological Awareness
Adult Direction	"Remove /s/ from *cats* and tell what is left."	"Look at these pictures. Point to the picture that shows what is left when you add /s/ to *cat.*"
Child Response	"Cat."	Among an array of three pictures (i.e., a group of cats, one cat, & a dog and cat), points to the picture showing a group of cats.

Word and Syllable Awareness

Word and Syllable awareness refers to the understanding that words are made up of syllables or beats (Walsh, 2002). This includes counting syllables, counting words, segmenting syllables, blending syllables, and deleting syllables. At the most advanced level, word and syllable awareness is the ability to manipulate word parts to create new words (e.g., moving the parts in the word *wallpaper* around to make the word *paperwall;* Walsh).

Rhyming

Every word can be divided into two sections: onset and rime. The **onset** consists of the sound(s) found prior to the first vowel sound in a word (Adams, 1990). The **rime** is made up of the sounds in the word that follow the onset. For example:

Word	Onset	Rime
cat	*c*	at
snap	*sn*	ap
jacket	*j*	acket

Rhyming refers to a person's skill in (1) recognizing words with similar rimes (i.e., rhyme identification) and (2) generating words that have identical rimes (i.e., rhyme production). Phonological awareness activities often contain tasks for both skills (e.g., "Which of these words rhymes with *snip: snap, step,* or *tip?*" and "Give a word that rhymes with *blink.*"

Phonological Processing

Phonological processing is not often discussed in literature that describes phonological awareness. However, it is critical to understand how this term relates to phonological awareness. Phonological processing refers to using phonological information to process oral and written language (Hodson & Edwards, 1997). The same phonological processing system children used to process spoken language when they were younger forms the foundation for their written language development (Pring & Snowling, 1986). When phonological processing for oral language is impaired and the child shows an expressive phonological disorder and phonological awareness deficits, reading and spelling difficulties are predictable (Stackhouse, 1997).

Phonics

Phonics is an instructional practice that shows the learner how written letters (i.e., graphemes) are related to speech sounds (i.e., phonemes). Phonics is also described as a systematic, structured, and hierarchical approach to teaching reading and writing. (Snow, Burns, & Griffin, 1998). Terms related to phonics include:

- **Graphemes**—The visual forms of speech sounds (a.k.a. letters)
- **Alphabetic principle**—The use of letters to represent speech sounds that combine to make words (Moats, 1995)
- **Decoding**—Deriving a pronunciation for a sequence of letters based on knowledge of letter-sound correspondence (Hall & Moats, 1999)

Language Disorder

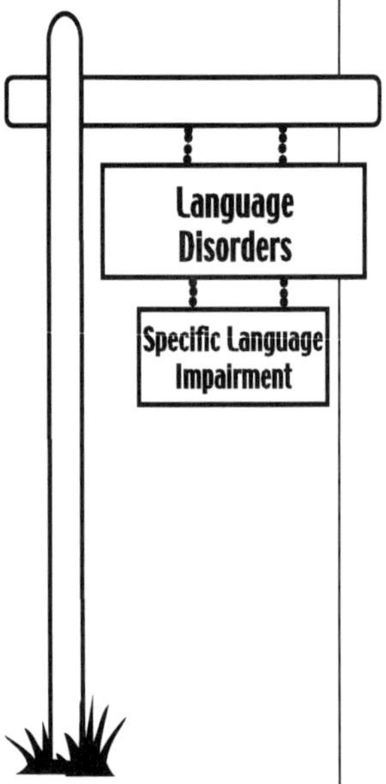

In the simplest terms, a **language disorder** is a difficulty understanding or using linguistic units, regardless of the environment (Nicolosi, Harryman, & Kresheck, 1996). A language disorder can be manifested in relation to content (e.g., vocabulary), form (e.g., syntax), and/or use (i.e., pragmatics) of language. A language disorder can be related to comprehension and/or production skills, including both oral and written forms.

Specific language impairment (SLI), a subtype of language disorder, is a deficit in language understanding and/or use with no evidence of neurological damage, hearing impairment, or delayed cognitive skills. That is, there is no known underlying condition. Therefore, it is a disability on the basis of exclusion (Leonard, 1991). Most children with a diagnosis of SLI have particular difficulty understanding and using grammar (Fey, Long, & Finestack, 2003).

Learning Disability

A **learning disability** is manifested by unexpected and unusual difficulty acquiring an academic skill (e.g., learning to decode for reading), when compared to the person's other abilities (e.g., solving math problems; Hall & Moats, 2000). Learning disabilities can be verbal, nonverbal, or both.

A **reading disability** is a subtype of learning disability in which a person has particular difficulty with comprehension of written language (Hall & Moats, 1999). It may include visual/orthographic difficulties, motivational deficit, attention problems, and/or language deficit (Catts, 2000). **Dyslexia** is a specific reading disability or language disorder manifested by difficulty in learning to read despite consistent and systematic instruction, adequate intelligence, and sociocultural opportunity (Catts, 2000).

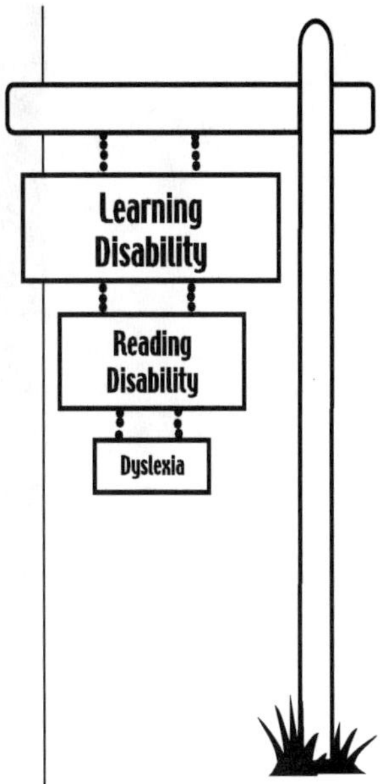

!Importance

The "chicken and the egg" debate typically results when educational professionals gather to discuss the relationship between phonological awareness, literacy, and the development of speech and language. Regardless of one's position on this complicated issue, it is recognized that phonological awareness skill is at least a piece of the literacy puzzle. A lack of phonological awareness skill may negatively impact reading and writing; weak reading and writing skills may result in reduced phonological awareness, or both relationships could be the case. It is also true that phonological awareness and speech-language skill are connected. While it is difficult to discern a cause-effect relationship between phonological awareness and speech and language development, research has found connections and offers suggestions for considering both in assessment and intervention.

Ignoring phonological awareness when assessing children, determining the need for intervention, and planning instruction is no longer an option. There is sufficient information to suggest strong connections among these skills. The following section describes these connections in greater detail and makes suggestions.

Relationship to Literacy

Literacy is an umbrella term that describes more than just reading and writing skills. The interrelated communicative processes of listening, speaking, reading, writing, and spelling comprise a complete picture of literacy (Silliman & Wilkinson, 1994). Thus, phonological awareness can promote or hinder literacy success as a part of this multifaceted communicative process.

So how does phonological awareness fit into the complicated process of becoming a successful reader? Scarborough (2001) suggests that during the course of becoming a skilled reader, 8 subskills are woven together into 2 major components—language comprehension and word recognition—that together make up the reading process (see Figure 1). Although the subskills are listed separately, they develop in an interactive fashion. In a skilled reader, language comprehension becomes increasingly more strategic and word recognition becomes increasingly more automatic (Scarborough, 2001). The lack of, or difficulty with, any of the subskills in Figure 1 can create challenges in the processes of (1) learning to read and (2) reading to learn—both important facets to literacy success.

Other researchers have found that strong readers have intact phonological awareness skills and that poor readers do not (Catts & Kamhi, 1999; Swank & Catts, 1994). In fact, Catts and Kamhi consider a deficiency in phonological

Figure 1 **Component Skills of Early Literacy Development**

Language Comprehension

- Background Knowledge (facts and concepts)
- Vocabulary (word knowledge and links)
- Language Structures (syntax/grammar)
- Verbal Reasoning (inference, metaphor, figurative language)
- Literacy Knowledge (print concepts, genrés)

Word Recognition

- **Phonological Awareness** (rhyme, syllables, and phonemes)
- Decoding (alphabetic principle)
- Sight Recognition (of common and familiar words)

→ **Skilled Reading** ←

Source: Scarborough (2001).

awareness to be the cause of some children's reading difficulties. The National Institutes of Health Council suggest that the single-best predictor of later reading skill is a child's phoneme segmentation skill as measured in 1st and 2nd grades (National Reading Panel, 2000).

Both reading and spelling require phonological awareness. Specifically, reading requires phoneme and syllable blending skills, while spelling is more closely dependent on segmentation skills (Ehri, 2000).

Improved phonological awareness skills have a positive impact on later literacy skills—that is, reading and writing (Blachman, 1994; Lundberg, Frost, & Peterson, 1988; O'Connor, Jenkins, Leicester, & Slocum, 1993; Warrick, Rubin, & Rowe-Walsh, 1993). Many reading difficulties appear to be preventable if at-risk children are provided with effective phonological awareness activities in preschool and kindergarten (Montgomery, 2001).

Relationship to Speech and Language Development

As mentioned, the question "Which came first?" can be posed concerning the influence of phonological awareness on speech and language development. Scarborough (2001) proposes a hybrid model to explain the connection between early speech and language development and later reading (dis)abilities. Likewise, a language disorder or learning disability can be explained by such a model, in which an underlying condition can cause harmful effects on one or on many skills, and in which one or more of the skills may affect another skill.

To better understand Scarborough's (2001) model, imagine a 7 year-old child who suffered from recurrent middle ear infections from 9 to 24 months of age. At age 7, this child may present with weak phonological awareness (e.g., does not rhyme and does not demonstrate phonemic awareness), several remaining articulation errors (e.g., distortion of /s/, /ʃ/, /ʧ/, /θ/, /ð/, /l/, and /r/), and delayed decoding skills as compared to peers. However, this same child may demonstrate age-appropriate vocabulary comprehension and background knowledge such that, aside from reading skill development, other academic skills are within normal limits for a child his or her age. The underlying condition (i.e., recurrent middle ear infections) may have negatively impacted the child's phonological awareness, decoding, and phonology, but may not have affected background knowledge or vocabulary comprehension skills. Furthermore, the deficient phonological awareness, decoding, and phonology may negatively impact each other.

A hybrid model can begin to explain inconsistencies in the profiles of students who struggle with one, some, or all of the speech and language skills that contribute to communication and literacy success. Language and speech (or phonology), can be positively or negatively influenced by a known or unknown underlying condition that is also influencing phonological awareness and other reading skills.

Communication skills, specifically phonology (speech production), can have a significant positive or negative impact on phonological awareness and consequently on reading skill. An intact speech-sound system organizes a child's phonological code; heightens the awareness of sounds in words; and, in turn, facilitates the acquisition of a graphemic code (Adams, 1990; Goldsworthy, 1998; Hodson, 2000). Accordingly, children with phonological disorders are at risk for reading difficulties (Fey, 1999). Research has shown that 50% of the words misspelled by children in grades 1–3 contain spelling errors that reflect the children's pronunciation errors or phonological process simplifications (Hoffman & Norris, 1989). Furthermore, remnants of a preschool phonological disorder, specifically reading and spelling difficulties, can frequently be seen throughout childhood and into adulthood (Lewis & Freebairn, 1992).

Preschool language status is an important variable when anticipating later reading and spelling performance (Lewis & Freebairn, 1992). A general understanding and use of language in kindergarten is the single best predictor of reading success in 2nd grade (Catts, Fey, Zhang, & Tomblin, 1999). Since language cannot be removed from the reading process, most children with reading difficulties also demonstrate language difficulties (Kamhi & Catts, 1991). In fact, 35–75% of children who exhibit a speech, language, and/or learning disability in early childhood will have difficulty learning to read (O'Keefe, 2000). In addition, there is frequently a lasting effect of preschool language disorder well into adolescence and adulthood (Lewis & Freebairn, 1992). Adolescents with histories of preschool speech and language disorders frequently demonstrate persistent communication, academic, and social difficulties (Lewis & Freebairn, 1992). Phonological awareness training with 4- and 5-year-old children with speech and/or language disorders has a significant and positive influence on speech production, language level, phonological awareness skills, reading skills, and writing skills (Gillon, 2000; van Kleeck, Gillam, & McFadden, 1998).

Speech-language pathologists are uniquely qualified to identify children who have weak phonological awareness skills, even before specific reading instruction begins (Catts, Fey, Zhang, & Tomblin, 2001). It is part of the scope of practice of clinicians to target phonological awareness skills in an attempt to prevent and/or treat reading and writing difficulties (ASHA, 2001) and to facilitate phonological development, so as to steer children towards literacy success (see Figure 2).

Figure 2

Influence of Weak/Strong Phonological Awareness Skills

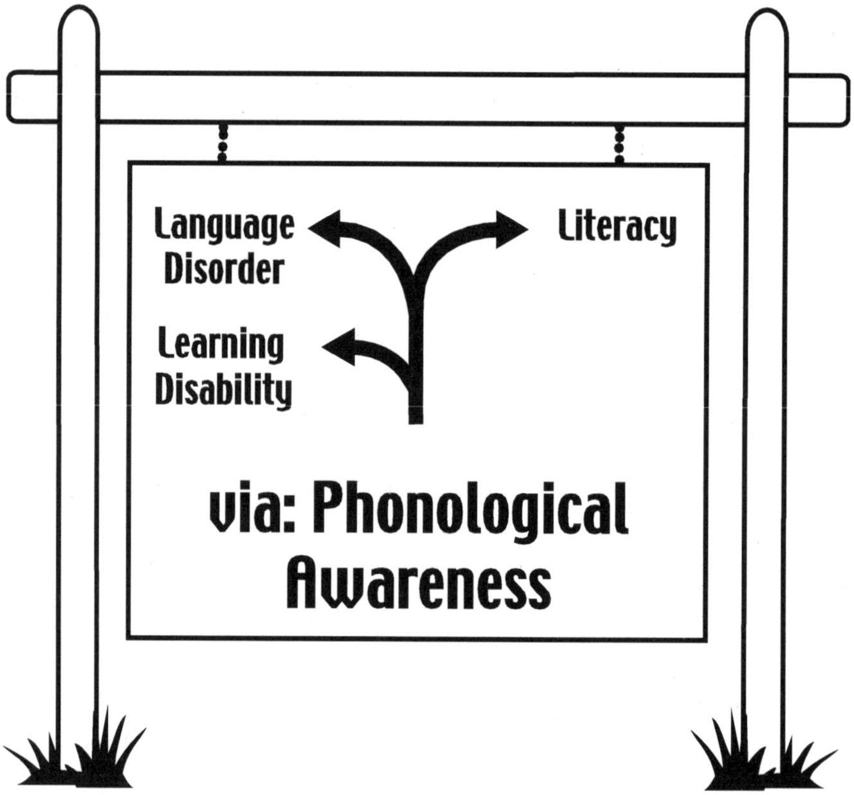

Development

Phonological awareness skills do not develop in a linear fashion. There is no "mastery" formula to suggest that children become proficient at one level of phonological awareness before developing the next level of skills. Phonological awareness skills develop like many other skills: with interplay between and among the various subskills and levels of difficulty. There are, however, some general stages of development. For the most part, phonological awareness skills tend to emerge as shown in Figure 3.

Figure 3 **Development of Phonological Awareness Skills**

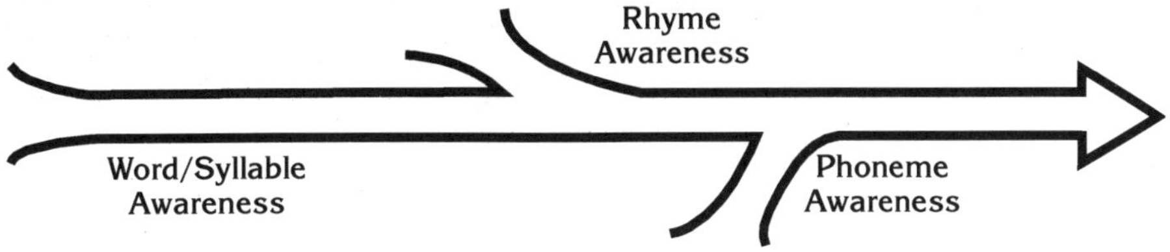

This progression does not dictate mastery of one skill before the next skill emerges. This distinction is critical. For example, research has shown that rhyme awareness and phoneme awareness can be unique constructs in some children and that the development of rhyme does not necessarily lead to the development of phonemic awareness skills (Martin & Byrne, 2002; Muter, Hulme, Snowling, & Taylor, 1998). To illustrate this point, Muter et al. (1998) found that phoneme segmentation skills, as evaluated at the end of 1st grade, showed a strong positive correlation to reading and spelling, while rhyming did not. However, when tested at the end of 2nd grade, rhyming showed a predictive effect on spelling, but not on reading. The 3 phonological awareness skill areas of word and syllable awareness, rhyme awareness, and phoneme awareness are described on the pages that follow.

Be Careful!

Word and Syllable Awareness

Since single words and syllables are relatively large units, they are more salient and easier to segment and blend than individual phonemes. Words can be created and divided based on their syllables. Segmentation of compound words (e.g., *baseball)* precedes segmentation of noncompound words (e.g., *Florida).* The developmental hierarchy of word and syllable awareness tasks (in order of emergence) is as follows:

➤ Playing with Words
↓
➤ Segmenting Syllables
↓
➤ Blending Syllables
↓
➤ Deleting Syllables
↓
➤ Manipulating Syllables

Table 2 (see page 19) provides descriptions, examples, and ages of emergence for each of these 5 word and syllable awareness subskills. This information can help guide instructional planning and assist with decisions of when to refer a child for more thorough assessment.

In addition to the general progression of subskills listed above, there are a few other developmental notes to consider. It is typically easier to add, delete, and/or manipulate final words and syllables than those in the initial and medial positions of sentences and words; likewise, the initial position is easier than the medial (O'Keefe, 2000). For example, it will probably be easier for a child to remove *ball* from the word *snowball,* than it will be for him or her to remove *side* from the word *sidewalk* (O'Keefe, 2000). Also, for syllable blending tasks, the longer the pause between the syllables, the more challenging the task.

Rhyme Awareness

The developmental hierarchy of rhyme awareness tasks (in order of emergence) is as follows:

- ➤ Spontaneously Producing Rhymes
  ↓
- ➤ Identifying Rhymes
  ↓
- ➤ Generating Rhymes
  ↓
- ➤ Judging Rhymes
  ↓
- ➤ Categorizing Rhymes

Table 2 (see page 19) provides descriptions, examples, and ages of emergence for each of these 5 rhyme awareness subskills. This information can help guide instructional planning and assist with decisions of when to refer a child for more thorough assessment.

In addition to the hierarchy above, rhyming tasks progress in difficulty based on the element of syllabicity. Rhymes for single-syllable words are easier to generate than rhymes for multisyllabic words. Children will first generate rhymes for words like *cat, bug,* and *ball.* As rhyming skill develops, and children fully understand the concept of rhyme, they become proficient at rhyming multisyllabic words like *under, sprinkle,* and *belly.*

Phoneme Awareness

Words and syllables can be created and divided based on their phonemes (i.e., sounds). Phoneme awareness (sometimes called *phonemic awareness)* often requires explicit and intense instruction, especially when considering children at-risk for reading difficulty (Catts, 1991). As phonemes are identified, segmented, blended, deleted, and manipulated, children demonstrate their awareness of how these discrete sounds form units of meaning and how meaning can change when phonemes change. Phoneme awareness is the highest level of phonological awareness and typically develops after word and syllable awareness and rhyme awareness have at least begun to emerge (Catts). The following is a developmental hierarchy (in order of emergence) of phonemic awareness subskills:

➤ Blending Phonemes
↓
➤ Segmenting Phonemes
↓
➤ Deleting Phonemes
↓
➤ Manipulating Phonemes

Table 2 provides descriptions, examples, and ages of emergence for each of these 4 phoneme awareness subskills. This information can help guide instructional planning and assist with decisions of when to refer a child for more thorough assessment.

In addition to the hierarchy suggested above, phoneme awareness tasks progress in difficulty based on sound features, word length, word and syllable shapes, and on the position of sounds in words. Unlike manipulating syllables or words, it is easier to delete and manipulate sounds in the initial position in words than in the medial and/or final positions (Stackhouse, 1997). Furthermore, a phoneme at the end of a word is easier to blend, segment, and manipulate than a phoneme in a medial position. Consonants are easier to segment, blend, delete, and manipulate than vowel sounds. Fricative sounds (e.g., /s/ and /f/) are easier than nonfricative sounds (e.g., /p/, /g/, and /t/) because they are more salient and easier to sustain as they are produced by holding the articulators in a steady position with a prolonged airstream (Content, Morais, Alegria, & Bertelson, 1982; Hubbard & Mahanna-Boden, 2000; Treiman & Baron, 1981). Postvocalic liquids (/1/ and /r/) and postvocalic nasals (/m/, /n/, and /ŋ/) are the most challenging phonemes to segment from words (Treiman, Zukowski, & Richmond-Welty, 1995). Logically, shorter words are easier to blend, segment, and rhyme than longer words. Also, Goswami & Bryant (1990) found that word and syllable shapes that include consonant blends (e.g., c*rust, clips, sink,* and *splits),* are more challenging when used in phonemic awareness tasks than those that include only consonant singletons and vowel sounds (e.g., *bag, hall,* and *sheep).* Finally, for phonemic blending tasks, the longer the pause between the phonemes, the more challenging the task.

Table 2

General Emergence of Phonological Awareness Skills

	Skill	Description	Example Task	Age of Emergence*
Word and Syllable Awareness	Playing with Words	Counting, tapping or clapping out the number of words in a phrase or sentence	"Clap 1 time for each word you hear in the sentence *The cat is playing*"	3–5 years
	Segmenting Syllables	Identifying each word in a compound word Identifying the syllables in words (e.g., clapping, tapping, or otherwise indicating each individual syllable)	"Tell me the 2 words in the compound word *cupcake*." "Touch 1 block for each beat you hear in the word *hamburger*."	4 years 4–5 years
	Blending Syllables	Stating the word formed when two or more segmented syllables are presented	"What word do you hear if you blend *can* and *dy*?"	4–5 years
	Deleting Syllables	Stating what remains when asked to remove one or more syllables from a given word	"Say *Tuesday*. Now say *Tuesday* without the *day*"	5 years
	Manipulating Syllables	Interchanging syllables in words to form new and/or nonsense words	"Put the *back* from *backpack* at the end of *under*"	7+ years
Rhyme Awareness	Spontaneously Producing Rhymes	Using rhyming words prior to the concept of rhyme being established	Child rattles off word strings like *"Fall, ball, mall"* but does not generate an answer when asked "What rhymes with *ball*?"	3–4 years
	Identifying Rhymes	Understanding that certain words "go together" because of matching ending sounds	"Do these words rhyme: *cat, fat*?"	4–5 years
	Generating Rhymes	Producing one or more rhymes for a given word	"Say a word that rhymes with *hug*."	5+ years
	Judging Rhymes	Comparing rhyming and nonrhyming words and identifying any rhyming matches Selecting a word that does not rhyme with a given set of words (i.e., an oddity task)	"Listen to these words and tell me which ones rhyme: *pen, when, tip*." "Listen to these words and tell me which one does not rhyme: *pen, when, tip*."	6–7 years 6–7 years
	Categorizing Rhymes	Sorting and grouping words based on rhyme families	Present a child with rhyming picture cards like *cat, book, hat, hook, cup, rat, pup,* then say, "Put pictures that rhyme into piles."	6–7 years

Continued on next page

Go-To Guide for Phonological Awareness © 2004 Thinking Publications
Duplication permitted for educational use only.

Table 2—*Continued*

	Skill	Description	Example Task	Age of Emergence*
Phoneme Awareness	Blending Phonemes	Stating the word formed when two or more segmented sounds are presented	"What word do you hear if you blend /d/, /ɔ/, /g/?"	6 years
	Segmenting Phonemes	Identifying the sounds in words (e.g., clapping, tapping, or otherwise indicating each sound)	"Clap 1 time for each sound you hear in the word *fan*."	6 years
	Deleting Phonemes	Stating what remains when asked to remove one or more sounds from a given word	"Say *house*. Now say *house* without the first sound."	7 years
	Manipulating Phonemes	Interchanging sounds in a word to form a new or nonsense word	"Say *bus*. Now say *bus* with a /d/ instead of a /s/ sound at the end."	7^+ years

Sources: Adams (1990); Blachman (1991); Bradley and Bryant (1983); Goldsworthy (1998); Perfetti (1995); Stackhouse (1997); Stanovich (1988); Torgesen (1999); van Kleeck (1998).

*Age of emergence applies to children with typical development.

Go-To Guide for Phonological Awareness © 2004 Thinking Publications
Duplication permitted for educational use only.

Assessment

If, during a complete assessment of a child's communicative or literacy development, it is determined that phonological awareness may be a factor, an assessment of phonological awareness should be undertaken. As with any assessment, an evaluation of phonological awareness skills should include a description of a child's present level of performance (PLOP), including identifying strengths and weaknesses, and should suggest the direction for intervention, if warranted. Appropriate attention must be paid to all aspects of language and literacy development so that well-planned and comprehensive intervention can be designed; phonological awareness is but one component of literacy.

Be Careful!

Both informal and formal procedures are available for evaluating a child's phonological awareness skills. Each type and its corresponding strengths and weaknesses are described in the sections that follow.

Informal Procedures

Informal assessment includes procedures that observe and describe a child's skills. Informal procedures can include:

- Inventories/Checklists
- Rubrics
- Anecdotal notes
- Student portfolios

What these methods have in common is that they are nonstandardized. Strengths and weaknesses of using informal measures of assessment are listed in the following chart:

Informal Assessment Procedures	
Strengths	**Weaknesses**
• Inexpensive • Can be customized for an individual child • Allow for instruction and experimentation during administration (e.g., check for stimulability and test out instructional options) • Useful for identifying both strengths and weaknesses • Useful for program planning	• Subjective • Not prescriptive • Can be time consuming to develop and use • Difficult to locate • Do not generate standardized scores sometimes required to determine eligibility for receiving speech-language services

Clearly, informal assessments alone are not sufficient for developing a complete understanding of a child's intervention needs. However, informal procedures, because of their flexible, detailed, and descriptive nature, can be extremely helpful when planning phonological awareness instruction. Refer to **Appendix A** for a *Phonological Awareness Checklist.* This form may be useful for large-group screening or as a pre-referral procedure. When using this check-list, observe and interact with the child to conduct the age-appropriate tasks. Indicate with a plus sign (+) when a child is observed using a skill, and use a minus sign (–) to show lack of the skill. Review the results and determine whether further assessment is warranted by comparing the child's age to the age of emergence of the screened skills.

For a more in-depth look at phonological awareness, **Appendix B** offers a *Phonological Awareness Inventory* that can be helpful for identifying strengths and weaknesses and for generating intervention objectives and methods. When conducting this inventory with a child, use a plus sign (+) to mark items the child performs correctly spontaneously, use an asterisk (*) to note items the child performs correctly with support (e.g., repetition of the item, demonstration with an additional example, or use of manipulatives), and a minus sign (–) to score items in error. Since this is an informal assessment procedure, there are no basals or ceilings. Nor are there any stringent guidelines for when to abandon a type of task. As a general rule of thumb, consider discontinuing a specific type of task once a child has made 3 consecutive errors. However, attempt each type of task, since children develop these skills in an inconsistent fashion. For example, just because a child has not mastered syllable awareness, does not mean he or she doesn't have emerging skills in rhyme awareness. When finished with the inventory, look through the results to select areas of need for a child. Select all skills within an appropriate age of emergence to target through intervention activities.

Be Careful!

Other informal measures of phonological awareness skills can be found in the following resources:

- *The Literacy Link* (2002), by Peggy S. Northrup, Eau Claire, WI: Thinking Publications.
- *The Phonological Awareness Profile* (1995), by Carolyn Robertson and Wanda Salter, East Moline, IL: LinguiSystems.
- *Phonological Awareness Success* (2002), by Sheila J. Walsh, Eau Claire, WI: Thinking Publications.

Formal Procedures

Formal assessment includes procedures that are standardized and norm-referenced. Strengths and weaknesses of formal measures are listed in the following chart:

Formal Assessment Procedures	
Strengths	**Weaknesses**
• Allow child to be compared to norms • Provide evidence of eligibility or exclusion • Are consistent, valid, and reliable	• Expensive • Administration is rigid • Frequently do not assist in generating intervention objectives • May not help discover intervention methods/strategies for a particular child • Time consuming to administer and interpret

Formal procedures for assessing phonological awareness skills have the advantage of comparing a child's performance to normative data. This information is helpful when eligibility criteria for entrance to or exit from an intervention program is required. There are a variety of standardized tools that measure phonological awareness skills. **Appendix C** includes a listing of some of these batteries and a summary of each.

Be Careful!

Keep in mind that phonological awareness is not recognized as a specific area of potential disability in order to qualify a child for special education services in the public schools. Thus, a child who undergoes formal assessment of phonological awareness in this setting has likely been referred in response to more global concerns (e.g., potential language disorder, potential learning disability, potential articulation or phonology disorder). For this reason, other types of formal and informal assessment measures besides those for phonological awareness should also be conducted. Regardless of whether they are formal or informal, assessment results that explain a child's phonological awareness skills can be used to create a more complete profile of the child and to suggest a more comprehensive plan for intervention.

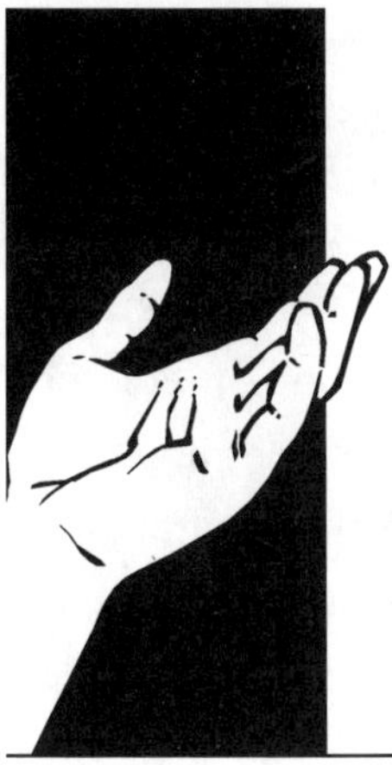

Intervention

Phonological awareness intervention is part of the scope of practice of a speech-language pathologist as suggested by the American Speech-Language-Hearing Association (ASHA; 2001). A variety of other educational professionals are also qualified to provide instruction in this area.

Phonological awareness skills can be improved through activities designed to target such skills (Adams, 1990; Blachman, 1989, 1994; Calfee, 1977; Torgesen, Wagner, & Rashotte, 1994). There are a multitude of commercially available instructional and intervention resources that, in whole or in part, target phonological awareness skills (see **Appendix D**). While many or most of these resources, activity kits, and guides are useful, instruction must be carefully planned, deliberate, and comprehensive. This section describes 4 characteristics of effective intervention, provides some basic guidelines for instruction, and explains the benefits of using children's literature in phonological awareness intervention.

Characteristics of Effective Intervention

Phonological awareness intervention must be:

- Explicit
- Systematic
- Supportive
- Intensive

These 4 characteristics are described in detail on the pages that follow.

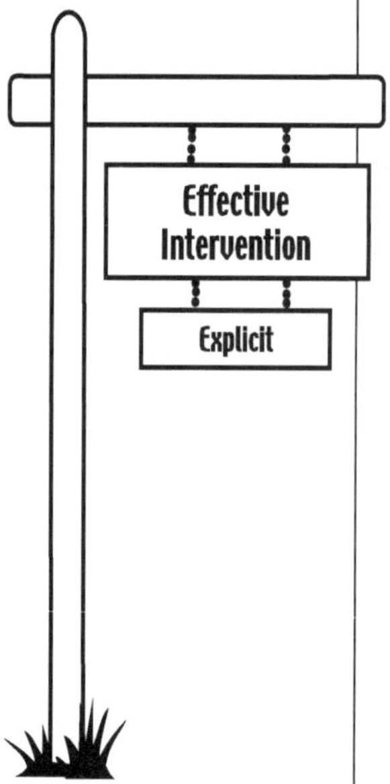

Explicit

Since phonological awareness skills do not develop naturally in some children, especially those with documented speech and/or language disorders, instruction of these skills must be explicit. Children may fail to acquire and/or apply phonological awareness skills unless instruction is unambiguous and mediated. Phonological awareness training is most effective when "meta" strategies are incorporated and children are presented with explanations of tasks and strategies, including statements of mediated learning (Blachman, 1991; Bradley & Bryant, 1983; Hodson, 2000). By mediating a child's learning through definite statements and questions (e.g., "I changed the first sound in the word in order to think of a rhyme" or "How did you figure out the number of sounds in that word?"), the educator focuses the child's attention on the salient features of a task. Mediated learning strategies and explicit statements increase the likelihood that skills will generalize to other situations and settings (Feuerstein, 1980).

The amount of explicitness that accompanies instruction will, and should, increase as the age of the child increases. For example, when working with a group of 4-year-olds on syllable segmentation skills, it is appropriate to introduce the task with a general statement such as the following:

> "Today we're going to play with words. We will be listening to lots of long words and clapping one time for each beat we hear in each word. Watch me do the first one."

However, when working with a group of 6-year-olds on phoneme deletion skills, instruction will be more explicit and include frequent statements of the way a skill is performed and the significance of the skill. For example:

> "We all know that words are made up of sounds. You have had lots of practice blending sounds together to make words and taking words apart to tell their sounds. Today we are going to practice taking away sounds from words and telling what is left. For example, I can say the word *hold* and then I can take away the last sound in *hold*, the /d/ sound. It turns into *hole*. Taking away the /d/ changed *hold* into *hole*. Let's try some more."

Whether implementing a customized plan or using a commercially available product, include an appropriate level of explicitness in each lesson so that children who struggle with these skills develop a better understanding of them and the rationale for their importance.

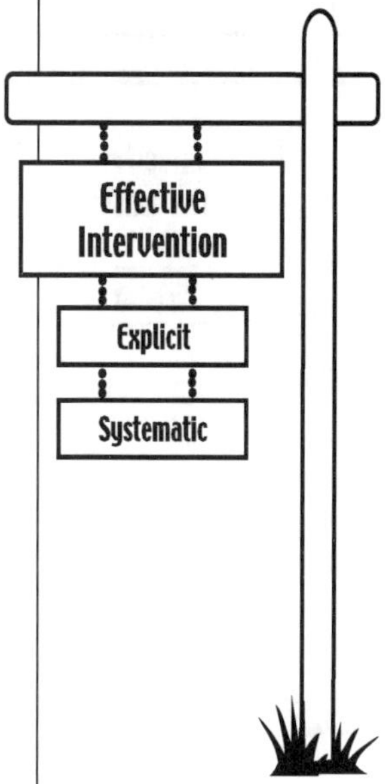

Systematic

Like all effective instruction, phonological awareness skills must be targeted systematically. Systematic intervention can be reflected in 3 ways:

1. **Systematic Choice of Skills:** Skills that typically develop earlier in children should be targeted before later developing skills. It is critical that educators know the scope and sequence of the skills being taught. This allows for a natural progression from a child's present level of performance (PLOP) to the desired goal of phonological awareness.

   Speech-language pathologists are uniquely qualified to target phonological awareness skills because of their knowledge of the development of speech-sound use, expressive and receptive language skills, and phonological awareness. Understanding the typical development of phonological awareness skills allows educators to establish an instructional plan that puts tasks into a reasonable order. Keep in mind that children do not need to master one type of phonological awareness skill in order to be ready for the next type of skill. Choose a group of skills that are within expectations of emergence and work back and forth between the skills. Refer to Table 2 (on pages 19–20) to assist with the development of a systematic plan for targeting phonological awareness skills.

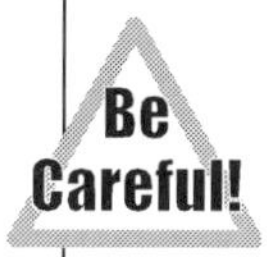

2. **Systematic Lesson Plan:** There must be a procedure for introducing a skill, providing explicit instruction (so that children understand the use of a skill), providing sufficient production-practice (so that children can develop their use of the skill), reviewing, and frequently assessing the performance of children. Constructing lesson plans in a systematic way to reflect this organization increases the likelihood that plans are comprehensive and that they offer the repetition, progression, and cohesion that contributes to skill acquisition and generalization.

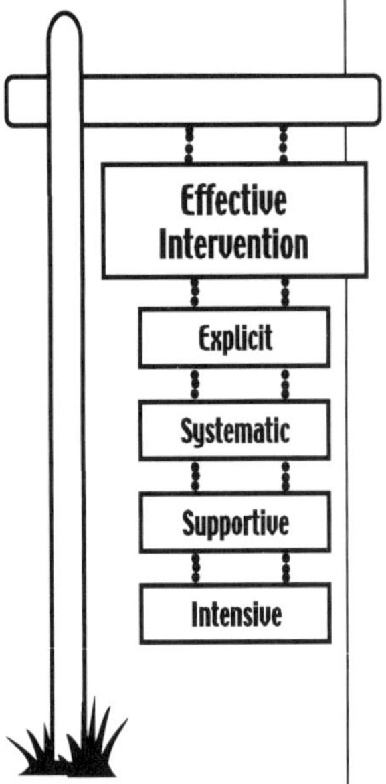

3. **Systematic Use of Support:** During the instruction and production-practice phases of a lesson, educators must have a system established for offering the appropriate amount and type of support and reinforcement to children. This will vary depending on the specific needs of individual children, but should incorporate moving from a high level of support and modeling to none. Consider the types of support discussed in the following section when designing a systematic plan for providing instruction, correction, and support to children working on phonological awareness skills.

Supportive

Supportive intervention provides scaffolded instruction as children are learning and practicing phonological awareness skills. Support must be systematically designed to move from a high level to a low level as needed and appropriate. The support can take the form of verbal, physical, visual, and gestural stimuli. Furthermore, the support needed for one child might be different than that needed for another child. It is important to be familiar and comfortable with the different options for providing support, so that they can be incorporated or removed whenever needed. Table 3 offers 6 ways to provide support (in varying degrees) for phonological awareness tasks. Depending on each specific skill and activity, other types of support may also be an option. It is important to look for unique and task-specific ways to provide support during activities. Enlisting the assistance of classroom teachers, paraprofessionals, and parents can provide added support.

Intensive

Phonological awareness intervention must be a frequent and consistent component in a child's educational program. Educators must be "relentless" in their use of phonological awareness work with children who are at-risk for reading difficulties (Catts, 2000). Research has shown that when using instructional methods that do not include phonological awareness tasks, only about 25% of children who have reading disabilities actually overcome their disability and become functional readers (Catts). Thus, the "relentless" attack on phonological awareness skills in an attempt to prevent later reading difficulties seems reasonable.

Table 3

Continuum of Support

Most Support → Least Support

Type of Support	Description	Example
Have Children Respond in Unison	This technique takes pressure off a single child. As children respond in unison, offer your response at an elevated volume so children can hear an appropriate answer. Consider using classroom amplification to make your voice stand out above the children's.	Say, "Let's say the rhyme pair *cat/rat* together. While we say the words, listen to how they sound the same at the end. All together now: *cat/rat"* [in unison].
Model the Target	Use more frequent modeling as children begin to learn a skill. Then reduce the modeling as children get comfortable with a skill. Have children model for each other, when appropriate.	Say, "*Watermelon* is a long word and *bug* is a short word. Listen to these 2 words: *caterpillar* and *car. Caterpillar* is a long word. It has 4 beats: *cat* • *er* • *pill* • *ar. Car* is a short word with just 1 beat: *car."*
Stress the Target in Your Speech	Use emphasis and variation of pitch, loudness, and intonation to help children see the phonological awareness skill being highlighted.	Say, "Listen to these words. Tell me which 2 rhyme: *red, book, head."* [Use an increased volume when saying the words *red* and *head.]*
Provide a Visual or Physical Cue	Use picture cards, tokens, blocks, and gestures to help children learn and practice phonological awareness skills.	Provide the child with 3 wooden blocks and say, "Look, the blocks can be the sounds in the word *fan."* Point to 1 block as you say each sound in *fan."* Then say, "Now you use these blocks to show me the sounds in *pig."*
Give a Choice	Rather than letting children struggle to come up with an answer (and to avoid giving them the answer), provide a choice between two or more options. The greater the number of options, the greater the challenge. In addition, pay attention to how the options differ to control the level of challenge.	Rather than asking, "What sound do *car, cat,* and *comb* all start with?" ask, "Do *car, cat,* and *comb* start with /s/ or with /k/?" Rather than asking, "Does *bug* rhyme with *beg* or with *hug?"* ask, "Does *bug* rhyme with *car* or with *hug?"* (since *car* and *hug* are greater contrasts than *beg* and *bug).*
Repeat the Error	Demonstrate an error, without calling negative attention to it. This technique can help a child identify and correct a response.	If a child says that *sun* ends with /p/, say "Listen closely: *sun, sun.* Does it sound like there is a /p/ at the end of *sun?"*

Intervention resources and programs suggest a variety of time guidelines for conducting phonological awareness training. However, as long as instruction appears as a noticeable and consistent feature in a child's education program, it is more likely to have a beneficial effect. As with many types of intervention, the more, the better. Overlearning and repeated practice are vital to improvement in phonological awareness.

Basic Guidelines for Intervention

Be Careful!

Clinicians must remember that phonological awareness tasks are oral/listening activities. Therefore, most of the time, children should not be expected to read words during these tasks, nor should they be expected to tell the letters that are used to make various sounds. That is not to suggest that words and letters should not be used or talked about. Expose children to the words and letters constantly, and draw reference to them whenever it seems appropriate. However, do not initially expect or ask children to read words, to name letters, or to describe sound-symbol correspondence statements. Be aware, however, that phonological awareness skills such as identifying sounds within words, or components of clusters, sharpen as children learn to read or have experience with sound-letter correspondence. Therefore, at the phonemic level, reading will help develop phonological awareness.

Be Careful!

When pronouncing isolated phonemes during phonological awareness tasks, do not use the letter names (e.g., *tee);* rather, produce the sound that the phoneme makes (e.g., /t/). This can be especially challenging for voiced phonemes, where the temptation to add a vowel sound when pronouncing the sound (e.g., /tʌ/) exists. It is important that the letter names not be used in place of the phoneme sounds.

Use of Children's Literature in Intervention

In addition to using card games, hands-on activities, worksheets, and oral exercises, using children's books for phonological awareness tasks provides an endless supply of engaging and functional stimuli. Children tend to be naturally attracted to books. For younger children (ages 3–8), colorful and amusing illustrations and the frequent use of rhythms, patterns, rhymes, and alliteration (i.e., repetition of the same initial sound [onset] in words) grabs their attention and keeps them focused on the oral expression of the language used in a story. For older children (ages 9–12), fun content and interesting characters can replace illustrations. These children continue to love rhythms, rhymes, patterns, and alliteration. Books with elements of alliteration and rhyme are perfect for exposing children to phonological awareness and providing practice using these skills. Moreover, a great number of classic children's books contain repetitive linguistic patterns, which give children increased opportunities for hearing and using a specifically selected target, whether it be phonological or linguistic. Finally, children's literature has the bonus feature of naturally eliciting conversation from children.

Using stories strategically with children certainly facilitates language development, speech development, phonological awareness skills, and an interest in reading and writing (Watson, Layton, Pierce, & Abraham, 1994). Norris and Hoffman (1993) found that written language, which is the basis of children's literature, is well-suited for facilitating the understanding and use of oral language (including phonological awareness skills) since written language is visual and contextualized, giving the child additional support for organizing concepts and skills.

Appendix E includes a listing of phonological awareness skills, a brief sampling of specific children's books that can be used to target each skill, and a sample dialogue. This appendix is provided to demonstrate how easily children's literature can be used to target phonological awareness skills. With very little extra planning, you can add great breadth to a language or literature lesson. Use this appendix as a springboard for using other books for phonological awareness fun.

Appendices

Phonological Awareness Checklist

Child's Name: ______________________________ Date: ______________

+/–	Skill/Task	Age of Emergence*
	Responds to and enjoys the rhythm and patterns of nursery rhymes, songs, and/or finger plays (e.g., joins in with motions and/or words, in unison)	2
	Responds appropriately to nursery rhymes or songs (e.g., completes a rhyme like "Pat-a cake, pat-a-cake, baker's man. Bake me a cake as fast as you ____")	3
	Spontaneously uses alliteration (e.g., can be overheard saying things like "*Bee, bay, by*")	3
	Claps out the syllables in 2-syllable compound words (e.g., responds when told to "Clap out the beats in *skateboard, bookshelf, backpack, doghouse, rowboat*")	4
	Demonstrates knowledge of long versus short words (e.g., can answer "Which word is long: *caterpillar* or *dog?*" or "Which word is short: *bee* or *bubblegum?*")	4
	Spontaneously uses simple rhymes (e.g., can be overheard saying things like "*Dog, log, sog, mog*" just for fun)	4
	Recognizes a rhyming word pair (e.g., can answer "Do *cat* and *bat* rhyme? Do *love* and *bus* rhyme? Do *bubble* and *trouble* rhyme?")	4
	Claps out the syllables in 2-syllable and 3-syllable noncompound words (e.g., responds when told to "Clap out the beats in *rainbow, candy, coffee, under, umbrella, camera, radio, computer*")	4 1/2
	Blends 2 syllables together to make a compound word (e.g., responds when asked "What word do you get if you blend *suit* and *case?*")	4 1/2
	Blends 2 and 3 syllables together to make noncompound words (e.g., responds when told to "Put *can* and *dy* together and tell the word" or "Put *un, der,* and *stand* together and tell the word")	4 1/2
	Labels words appropriately as "long" or "short" (e.g., answers "Is *bug* a long word or a short word? How about *hi? Elevator? Fish? Operation?*")	4 1/2
	Deletes syllables from multisyllabic words and tells what remains (e.g., responds to "Take *pet* away from *carpet* and tell what is left" or "Take *sha* away from *shadow* and tell what is left")	5

Go-To Guide for Phonological Awareness © 2004 Thinking Publications
Duplication permitted for educational use only.

+/–	Skill/Task	Age of Emergence*
	Tells a word that rhymes with a given single-syllable word (e.g., responds to "Tell a word that rhymes with *sun.* With *face.* With *gum.* With *rat.* With *kick")*	5
	Tells a word that rhymes with a given two-syllable word (e.g., responds to "Tell a word that rhymes with *candy.* With *hello.* With *tower.* With *baby.* With *mixing")*	5
	Tells 3 words that rhyme with a given single-syllable word (e.g., answers when told to "Tell 3 words that rhyme with *day.* With *try.* With *bee")*	5½
	Identifies a word that does not rhyme with a given set of words (e.g. responds to "Listen: *Hat, cat, car, mat.* Which word does not rhyme?")	6
	Blends 3 phonemes to make a word (e.g., answers "What word do you get if you blend /p/, /ɛ/, /n/; /f/, /eɪ/, /s/; /l/, /ɪ/, /p/; /s/, /i/, /d/?")	6
	Tells the first sound in a given word (e.g., answers "What sound does *house* start with? How about *mud? Cup? Sugar? Paper? Flower? Stick?")*	6
	Tells 2 or more words that start with a given sound (e.g., answers when told to "Tell 2 words that start with /s/. How about /f/, /p/, /t/, /r/, /ʃ/?")	6
	Manipulates syllables to form new words (e.g., responds to "Put *rain* from *rainbow* at the end of the word" or "Put *fall* from *waterfall* at the beginning of the word")	6–7
	Segments 3- and 4-phoneme words to tell the sounds (e.g., responds to "Break apart the sounds in the word *fan.* Now try *red. Face. Cake. Bed. Baby. Heart. Farm")*	7
	Tells the final sound in a given word (e.g., answers "What sound does *case* end with? How about *dog? Light? Frame? Rabbit? Chocolate? Hats?")*	7
	Tells 2 or more words that end with a given sound (e.g., answers when told to "Tell 2 words that end with /s/. How about /f/, /p/, /t/, /r/, /ʃ/?")	7
	Deletes initial and final sounds from words and tells what remains (e.g., responds to "Take the /m/ away from *man* and tell what is left. Now take the /p/ away from *peel.* Take the /t/ away from *hat")*	7
	Tells the medial sound in words (e.g., responds to "Tell the middle sound in the word *meet.* How about *fry? Radio? Puppet? Woman?")*	7^+
	Blends 4^+ phonemes to make a word (e.g., answers "What word do you get if you blend /p/, /ɛ/, /n/, /i/ or /f/, /a/, /r/, /m/?")	7^+
	Manipulates initial and final sounds in words to make new words (e.g., responds to "Say *fish.* Now say it with a /w/ instead of a /f/" or "Say *back.* Now say it with a /d/ instead of a /k/")	7^+

Sources: Adams (1990); Blachman (1991); Bradley and Bryant (1983); Goldsworthy (1998); Perfetti (1995); Stackhouse (1997); Stanovich (1988); Torgesen (1999); van Kleeck (1998).

*Age of emergence applies to children with typical development

Go-To Guide for Phonological Awareness © 2004 Thinking Publications
Duplication permitted for educational use only.

Phonological Awareness Inventory

Child's Name: ______________________________ Date: ____________ Age: _____

Scoring Instructions

In each blank, write (+) to mark items the child performs correctly spontaneously, use a (*) to note items the child performs correctly with support (e.g., repetition of the item, demonstration with an additional example, or use of manipulatives), and a (–) to score items in error. There are no basals or ceilings and no stringent guidelines for discontinuing a task. Consider discontinuing a specific type of task once a child has made 3 consecutive errors. However, attempt each type of task. When finished with the inventory, look through the results to select areas of need for a child. Select all skills within an appropriate age of emergence to target through intervention activities.

Word Awareness

A. "Listen carefully. How many words do you hear?"

____ *Sam is mad.* (3)   ____ *The cat drank milk.* (4)

____ *An elephant is very big.* (5)   ____ *It is dark outside at night.* (6)

B. "Listen to each word pair. Say 'same' if both words sound the same. Say 'different' if the words sound different from each other."

____ *dog, bird*   ____ *cat, cat*   ____ *hello, help*   ____ *radio, radio*

Syllable Segmentation

A. "Listen carefully. After I say a word, you say the word and clap 1 time for each beat. For example, if I say, '***elephant,***' you would say, '***el*** (clap), ***e*** (clap), ***phant*** (clap).' ***Elephant*** has 3 claps. Now try these."

____ *fish* (1)   ____ *cupcake* (2)   ____ *rainbow* (2)   ____ *snowman* (2)

____ *umbrella* (3)   ____ *candy* (2)   ____ *elevator* (4)   ____ *camping* (2)

____ *computer* (3)   ____ *pan* (1)   ____ *alligator* (4)   ____ *tomato* (3)

 © 2004 Thinking Publications
Duplication permitted for educational use only.

B. "The word ***watermelon*** is a long word. It has 4 claps: ***Wa*** (clap), ***ter*** (clap), ***mel*** (clap), **on** (clap). ***Bug*** is a short word. It has 1 clap: ***bug*** (clap). Listen to each word. Tell if the word is long or short."

___ *eye* (short) ___ *telephone* (long) ___ *elevator* (long)

___ *page* (short) ___ *shark* (short) ___ *operation* (long)

___ *understanding* (long) ___ *card* (short) ___ *game* (short)

C. "Listen to the word ***cupcake.*** I hear 2 little words, ***cup*** and ***cake.*** Tell me the little words you hear in these big words."

_________ _________ *toothbrush* _________ _________ *tiptoe*

_________ _________ *snowman* _________ _________ *cowboy*

_________ _________ *shoelace* _________ _________ *bedtime*

Rhyme Awareness

A. "Listen to these words: ***rat, mat, hat.*** These words go together because they rhyme. Listen again: ***rat, mat, hat.*** These words rhyme because the last parts are the same. Listen to each set of words and tell if they rhyme."

___ *book, look* ___ *trust, crust* ___ *car, dog* ___ *pot, pet*

___ *toot, boot* ___ *blue, pie* ___ *wall, small* ___ *candy, dandy*

B. "Tell a word that rhymes with each word I say." Transcribe the child's responses in order to detect a pattern, if any. *[For increased challenge, ask the child to tell two words that rhyme with each given word.]*

___ *no* _______________ ___ *top* _______________ ___ *hug* _______________
response response response

___ *bed* _______________ ___ *cast* _______________ ___ *jelly* _______________
response response response

Go-To Guide for Phonological Awareness © 2004 Thinking Publications
Duplication permitted for educational use only.

C. "Listen to this group of words: ***run, fun, bun, chair*** and ***sun.*** In this group, the words ***run, fun, bun,*** and ***sun*** all go together because they rhyme. ***Chair*** does not go in that rhyming group. Now you tell the rhyming words in each group."

______________________ *head, red, sick, bed*

______________________ *me, up, tree, sea*

______________________ *blue, ball, tall, wall, call*

______________________ *eight, kite, hug, fight, right*

Syllable Blending, Deleting, and Manipulating

A. "If I put together ***skate*** and ***board,*** I get the word ***skateboard.*** Listen to these word parts. Put them together to make bigger words."

[Use a 2-second pause between each syllable.]

____ *dog • house* ____ *back • pack* ____ *row • boat*

____ *un • der • stand* ____ *cal • en • dar* ____ *up • side • down*

[Use a 4-second pause between each syllable.]

____ *pe • nny* ____ *wo • man* ____ *wea • ther*

____ *bas • ket • ball* ____ *to • ma • to* ____ *ther • mom • e • ter*

B. "It's fun to play with words and make new words by taking parts away. Listen. I can say ***airplane*** without ***air*** and it would be ***plane.*** If I say ***funny*** without ***fun,*** it would be ***knee.*** Try these."

____ Say ***shoelace.*** Now say ***shoelace*** without ***shoe.*** *(lace)*

____ Say ***rainbow.*** Now say ***rainbow*** without ***rain.*** *(bow)*

____ Say ***waterfall.*** Now say ***waterfall*** without ***fall.*** *(water)*

____ Say ***sleeping.*** Now say ***sleeping*** without ***ing.*** *(sleep)*

____ Say ***purple.*** Now say ***purple*** without ***pur.*** *(ple)*

____ Say ***hamburger.*** Now say ***hamburger*** without ***ham.*** *(burger)*

____ Say ***calculator.*** Now say ***calculator*** without ***tor.*** *(calcula)*

____ Say ***computer.*** Now say ***computer*** without ***pu.*** *(comter)*

 © 2004 Thinking Publications
Duplication permitted for educational use only.

C. "Sometimes it's fun to move around the parts in words. I can say the word ***waterfall,*** and then I can put the ***fall*** in front of the ***water*** and say ***fallwater.*** Now you try these."

____ Say ***flashlight.*** Now put the ***flash*** after the ***light*** and what do you get? *(lightflash)*

____ Say ***windshield.*** Now put the ***shield*** before the ***wind*** and what do you get? *(shieldwind)*

____ Say ***grasshopper.*** Now put the ***grass*** after the ***hopper*** and what do you get? *(hoppergrass)*

D. "Listen to these words: ***tool, pool, car.*** The word that does not rhyme in this group is ***car. Tool*** and ***pool*** rhyme. Now listen to each group of words and tell the 1 that does not rhyme with the others."

____ *car, far, boat*

____ *baby, maybe, ladder*

____ *meet, store, feet, seat*

____ *dog, kite, fight, light*

____ *pen, cow, hen*

____ *candy, carpet, handy*

Phoneme Awareness

A. "Listen to these sounds: /b/ • /ɛ/ • /d/. Blended together, /b/ • /ɛ/ • /d/ says ***bed.*** Listen to these sets of sounds. Blend each set together and tell the word." *[Use a 1- or 2-second pause between each sound.]*

____ /ʌ/ • /p/ *(up)*

____ /n/ • /aɪ/ • /n/ *(nine)*

____ /w/ • /ɪ/ • /n/ • /ɚ/ *(winner)*

____ /p/ • /o/ • /t/ • /e/ • /t/ • /o/ *(potato)*

____ /d/ • /æ/ • /d/ *(dad)*

____ /l/ • /e/ • /d/ • /i/ *(lady)*

____ /b/ •/r/ • /ɛ/ • /d/ *(bread)*

Go-To Guide for Phonological Awareness © 2004 Thinking Publications
Duplication permitted for educational use only.

B. "The first sound in the word ***house*** is /h/. Tell the first sound you hear in each word."

____ *ball* ____ *goat* ____ *thumb* ____ *green* ____ *sun* ____ *happy*

C. "The words ***pig, pencil,*** and ***puppy*** all start with /p/. Tell 2 words that start with each sound." Record responses to detect any patterns and to reveal real vs. nonsense words.

____ /k/ ______________ ____ /j/ ______________ ____ /r/ ______________
______________ ______________ ______________

____ /f/ ______________ ____ /m/ ______________ ____ /d/ ______________
______________ ______________ ______________

____ /h/ ______________ ____ /o/ ______________ ____ /v/ ______________
______________ ______________ ______________

D. "Listen carefully. After I say a word, you say the word and clap 1 time for each sound. For example, if I say '***cook,***' you would say '***c*** (clap), ***oo*** (clap), ***k*** (clap).' Cook has 3 claps. Now try these."

____ *two* (2) ____ *odd* (2) ____ *cup* (3)

____ *red* (3) ____ *foot* (3) ____ *zip* (3)

____ *cookie* (4) ____ *candy* (5) ____ *crust* (5)

E. "The last sound in the word ***black*** is /k/. Tell the last sound you hear in each word."

____ *pot* ____ *snack* ____ *bus* ____ *tall*

____ *wish* ____ *pups* ____ *clown* ____ *puppet*

F. "The words ***bat, cat,*** and ***rat*** all end with the /t/ sound. Tell 1 word that ends with each sound." Record responses to detect any patterns and to reveal real vs. nonsense words.

____ /g/ ______________ ____ /ʃ/ ______________ ____ /d/ ______________

____ /v/ ______________ ____ /m/ ______________ ____ /s/ ______________

____ /k/ ______________ ____ /o/ ______________ ____ /p/ ______________

 © 2004 Thinking Publications
Duplication permitted for educational use only.

G. "I can say the word ***book*** without the /b/ sound. It would be ***ook.*** Now you try saying these words without certain sounds."

____ Say ***door.*** Now say ***door*** without the /d/ sound. *(or)*

____ Say ***pod.*** Now say ***pod*** without the /d/ sound. *(pa)*

____ Say ***sand.*** Now say ***sand*** without the /d/ sound. *(san)*

____ Say ***happy.*** Now say ***happy*** without the /h/ sound. *(appy)*

____ Say ***part.*** Now say ***part*** without the /p/. *(art)*

____ Say ***trap.*** Now say ***trap*** without the /t/. *(rap)*

____ Say ***funny.*** Now say ***funny*** without the ending sound. *(fun)*

____ Say ***trace.*** Now say ***trace*** without the beginning sound. *(race)*

H. "The middle sound in the word ***seed*** is /i/. You tell me the middle sound in each of these words."

____ *dry* ____ *stacks* ____ *peel* ____ *kit*

I. "Sometimes it's fun to move around the sounds in words. I can say the word ***fish,*** or I can use a /w/ sound instead of a /f/ sound and change it to the word ***wish.*** Now you try these."

____ Say ***two.*** Now add a /n/ sound at the end of ***two.*** *(tune)*

____ Say ***eye.*** Now add a /p/ sound at the beginning of ***eye.*** *(pie)*

____ Say ***sun.*** Now use a /f/ sound instead of a /s/ sound. *(fun)*

____ Say ***kitten.*** Now use a /m/ sound instead of a /k/ sound. *(mitten)*

____ Say ***love.*** Now use a /k/ sound instead of a /v/ sound. *(luck)*

____ Say ***hut.*** Now use an /æ/ sound instead of an /ʌ/ sound. *(hat)*

Comments / Patterns / Intervention Ideas

Go-To Guide for Phonological Awareness © 2004 Thinking Publications
Duplication permitted for educational use only.

Phonological Awareness Formal Assessment Batteries

Test and Publisher Information	Age Range	Skills Assessed
Assessment of Sound Awareness and Production (ASAP) L. Mattes (2000) Available from: Academic Communication Associates 1–888–758–9558 *www.acadcom.com*	3+ Years	• Identifying Rhyming Words • Identifying Initial Sounds • Identifying Final Sounds • Describing the Location of Sounds in Words • Blending Sounds • Identifying Syllables • Using Sound Cues
Comprehensive Test of Phonological Processing (CTOPP) R. Wagner, J. Torgesen, and C. Rashotte (1999) Available from: Pro-Ed 1–800–897–3202 *www.proedinc.com*	5–24 Years	• Phoneme Deletion (Elision) • Rapid Color Naming • Blending Words • Sound Matching • Rapid Object Naming • Memory for Digits • Nonword Repetition • Blending Nonwords
Lindamood Auditory Conceptualization Test (LAC) C. Lindamood and P. Lindamood (1971) Available from: Pro-Ed 1–800–897–3202 *www.proedinc.com*	All Ages	• Phoneme Discrimination • Phoneme Segmentation
Phonemic-Awareness Skills Screening (PASS) L. Crumrine and H. Lonegan (2000) Available from: Pro-Ed 1–800–897–3202 *www.proedinc.com*	Grades 1–2	• Rhyme • Sentence Segmentation • Blending • Syllable Segmentation • Deletion • Phoneme Isolation • Phoneme Segmentation • Phoneme Substitution

Test and Publisher Information	Age Range	Skills Assessed
The Phonological Abilities Test V. Muter, C. Hulme, and A. Snowling (1997) Available from: The Psychological Corporation 1-800-872-1726 *www.psychcorp.com*	5–7 Years	• Rhyme Detection • Rhyme Production • Word Completion (Syllables & Phonemes) • Phoneme Deletion (Beginning/Ending)
The Phonological Awareness Test C. Robertson and W. Salter (2000) Available from: LinguiSystems 1-800-776-4332 *www.linguisystems.com*	5–9 Years	• Rhyme Discrimination & Production • Sentence/Syllable/Phoneme Segmentation • Phoneme Isolation (Initial/Medial/Final) • Syllable & Phoneme Deletion • Phoneme Substitution • Syllable & Phoneme Blending • Grapheme Identification • Decoding
Pre-Literacy Skills Screening (PLSS) L. Crumrine and H. Lonegan (2000) Available from: Pro-Ed 1-800-897-3202 *www.proedinc.com*	PreK–K	• Rhyming • Rapid Naming • Sentence Segmentation • Syllable Segmentation • Multisyllabic Word Repetition • Sentence Repetition • Blending • Letter Naming • Deletion
Test of Phonological Awareness (TOPA) J. Torgesen and B. Bryant (1994) Available from: Pro-Ed 1-800-897-3202 *www.proedinc.com*	Grade K–2	• Discrimination of Initial Sounds in Words (Kindergarten) • Discrimination of Final Sounds in Words (Grades 1–2)
Test of Phonological Awareness Skills (TOPAS) P. Newcomer and E. Barenbaum (2003) Available from: Pro-Ed 1-800-897-3202 *www.proedinc.com*	5–10 Years	• Rhyming • Incomplete Words • Phoneme Sequencing • Phoneme Deletion

Phonological Awareness Intervention Resources

Resource and Publisher Information	Age Range	Skills Targeted	Activity Format
The Animated-Alphabet Story, Song, and Action Book J. Stone (1998) Available from: J. Stone Creations 1–619-465-8278 *www.thinkingpublications.com*	PreK–Grade 3	• Recognizing Sounds • Recognizing Letters • Sound-Letter Correspondence	• Multisensory activities to help children sing, draw, gesture, and say sounds and letter names • 43 songs
Earobics Cognitive Concepts (1997) Available from: Thinking Publications 1–800–225–4769 *www.thinkingpublications.com*	4–7 Years *(Step 1)* 7–11 Years *(Step 2)* 11 Years–Adult *(Earobics 1)*	• Auditory Attention & Memory • Sound-Symbol Correspondence • Phoneme Discrimination/ Identification • Phoneme Segmentation • Phoneme Blending • Rhyming • Syllable Segmentation • Syllable Blending	• Computer program • 6 games and 309 levels *(Step 1* and *Earobics 1)* • 5 games and 593 levels *(Step 2)* • Home-use version available
I'm All Ears F. Avni and N. Schimmel (1999) Available from: Sister's Choice Recordings and Books 1-510-524-5804 *www.thinkingpublications.com*	4–7 Years	• Rhyme Recognition & Production • Syllable Segmentation & Deletion • Alliteration • Phoneme Segmentation & Deletion • Phoneme Manipulation	• Audio CD (or cassette) and a music/activity book that introduce and reinforce phonological awareness • 23 songs
Lindamood Phoneme Sequencing Program *(LiPS)* P. Lindamood and P. Lindamood (1998) Available from: Pro-Ed 1–800–897–3202 *www.proedinc.com*	K–Grade 3	• Phoneme Awareness • Phoneme-Sequencing • Beginning Reading Instruction	• Kit including manipulatives, step-by-step procedures, scripted examples, and sample activities to promote metacognitive phonemic awareness

Resource and Publisher Information	Age Range	Skills Targeted	Activity Format
The Literacy Link P. Northrup (2002) Available from: Thinking Publications 1-800-225-4769 *www.thinkingpublications.com*	K–Grade 3	• Rhyming • Initial Consonant Identification • Learning Word Families • Phoneme Blending • Phoneme Segmentation • Phoneme-Grapheme Correspondence	• Book that teaches children hand symbols for 29 sounds to strengthen their sound-letter associations • 27 phonological awareness activities
More Story Making! R. Jones and C. DeBoer (2000) Available from: Thinking Publications 1-800-225-4769 *www.thinkingpublications.com*	PreK–Grade 3	• Counting Words in Sentences • Generating Rhyming Words • Counting Syllables in Words • Blending Syllables • Segmenting Words into Parts • Matching Initial/Medial/Final Sounds • Manipulating Sounds in Words	• Book exposing children to repetitive linguistic and phonological patterns as they create storybooks and participate in hands-on language activities • 47 pattern books
Phonemic Awareness Sound by Sound A. Peterson (2001) Available from: Academic Communication Associates 1-888-758-9558 *www.acadcom.com*	5–9 Years	• Sound Substitution • Sound Addition • Sound Deletion • Rhyme Production • Sound Manipulation	• Worksheet activities for phonological awareness training
Phonological Awareness Skills Program (PASP) J. Rosner (2002) Available from: Pro-Ed 1-800-897-3202 *www.proedinc.com*	Grades 1–5	• Phonological Awareness	• Test to identify needs • "Curriculum" to target phonological awareness skills
Phonological Awareness Success S. Walsh (2002) Available from: Thinking Publications 1-800-225-4769 *www.thinkingpublications.com*	4–9 Years	• Syllable Segmenting & Blending • Rhyme Identification & Production • Phoneme Segmenting & Blending • Whole-Word Segmentation	• Book of hands-on activities for children to learn and practice phonological awareness skills • 65 activities

Resource and Publisher Information	Age Range	Skills Targeted	Activity Format
Picture-Based Phonological Awareness Resource Academic Communication Associates (2003) Available from: Academic Communication Associates 1-888-758-9558 *www.acadcom.com*	5–10 Years	• Rhyming • Identifying/Matching Initial Sounds • Modifying Sounds to Create Words • Identifying Consonant/ Vowel Changes	• Picture games, picture cards, and worksheets
Silly Sounds Playground N. McKinley, L. Schreiber, A. Sterling-Orth, and S. Tobalsky (1999) Available from: Thinking Publications 1-800-225-4769 *www.thinkingpublications.com*	5–10 Years	• Segmenting Syllables • Blending Syllables • Blending Sounds • Manipulating Sounds • Rhyming (recognition and generation) • Segmenting Sounds	• Board game activity • 6 card decks
Sound Effects C. C. Spector (1999) Available from: Thinking Publications 1-800-225-4769 *www.thinkingpublications.com*	Grades 3–12	• Segment Words • Recognize Rhymes • Manipulate Sounds • Blend Sounds	• Book of jokes and riddles to help students identify, reflect on, and explain phonological awareness elements
Sounds Abound H. Catts and T. Olsen (2000) Available from: LinguiSystems 1-800-776-4332 *www.linguisystems.com*	4–9 Years	• Sound Awareness • Rhyming • Beginning & Ending Sounds • Segmenting & Blending Sounds • Matching Sounds with Letter Names	• Worksheet activities • 190 pages
Sounds Abound Storybook Activities S. Lachance (2002) Available from: LinguiSystems 1-800-776-4332 *www.linguisystems.com*	4–7 Years	• Word Awareness • Rhyming • Syllable Awareness • Sound Awareness	• Specified phonological awareness activities for 43 children's books • 233 pages

Resource and Publisher Information	Age Range	Skills Targeted	Activity Format
The Sounds Abound Program O. Lenchner and B. Podhajski (1998) Available from: LinguiSystems 1-800-776-4332 *www.linguisystems.com*	4–8 Years	• Sound Awareness • Rhyming • Beginning & Ending Sounds • Segmenting & Blending Sounds • Matching Sounds with Letter Names	• Pictures, songs, and games for phonological awareness practice • Manual, 195 illustrated cards, video
Sound Wizard O. Lenchner (2001) Available from: Thinking Publications 1-800-225-4769 *www.thinkingpublications.com*	5–9 Years	• Rhyme Recognition & Production • Syllable Segmentation & Deletion • Syllable Blending • Sound Identification & Matching • Sound Segmentation & Blending • Sound-Symbol Correspondence • Sound Manipulation	• 18 strategy-based card games • 6 large card decks and additional manipulatives
Sourcebook of Phonological Awareness Activities (Vol. 1 & 2) C. Goldsworthy (2001) Available from: Delmar Learning 1-800-998-7498 *www.delmarlearning.com*	Grades 1–5	• Word Awareness • Syllable Awareness • Phoneme Awareness	• Book that uses classic children's stories to emphasize and teach phonological awareness skills
Working Out with Phonological Awareness L. Schreiber, A. Sterling-Orth, S. Thurs, and N. McKinley (2000) Available from: Thinking Publications 1-800-225-4769 *www.thinkingpublications.com*	5–10 Years	• Segmenting Syllables • Blending Syllables • Blending Sounds • Manipulating Sounds • Rhyming • Segmenting Sounds • Working with Sound Clusters	• Activity book containing ready-to-use exercises • 50 Workouts (350 exercises)

Using Children's Literature to Teach Phonological Awareness

Syllable Awareness

Ages 3–8

From Head to Toe

(1997) by Eric Carle, New York: HarperTrophy

As each new animal is discovered in the book, model and help children clap, tap, or otherwise indicate each syllable in each animal's name (or for each word in a sentence, if working on word awareness instead of syllable awareness). For example:

> "This page says, 'I am an elephant and I can stomp my foot.' That gray elephant is big, and so is the word *elephant*. Let's clap 1 time for each beat in the word while we say *elephant. El • e • phant [said while clapping or holding up 1 finger for each syllable]*. How many beats are in that word?" *[Give children time to generate a response.]* "That's right, 3 beats. Let's clap it out again."

Ages 9–12

Charlotte's Web

(1952) by E.B. White, New York: HarperCollins

After each new character is introduced in the story, have students quickly sketch each character and segment the character's body into the number of syllables in his or her name. For example:

> "We met the rat Templeton in this chapter. Take 3 minutes to draw a picture of what you think Templeton, the grouchy rat on the farm, might look like. *[Wait until students have drawn the character.]* Great. Now think about Templeton's name: *Tem • ple • ton*. How many beats does his name have?" *[Give students time to generate a response.]* "That's right, 3 beats. Now take your pencil and divide your drawing into 3 sections, 1 for each part of Templeton's name." *[If desired, have students write Templeton's name on their drawings, dividing the name into syllables.]*

Rhyme Awareness

Ages 3–8

Don't Forget the Bacon
(1976) by Pat Hutchins, New York: Scholastic

For each funny phrase that rhymes with a phrase in the original shopping list that the mother gives her son in the beginning of the story, help children think of 1 or more additional rhyming phrases. For example:

> "Uh, oh. His mom said, *'a pound of pears'* but he is thinking it is *'a flight of stairs.'* That is funny because *pears* and *stairs* rhyme. Let's think of some more funny things that rhyme with 'a pound of pears' for his shopping list. Maybe *'nine long, blonde hairs'* or *'a room full of chairs.'* Now think of more." *[Give children time to generate responses.]* "That's great. *Bears* rhymes with *pears,* so *'a family of bears'* would be a great idea. Wouldn't it be funny to try to buy a family of bears at the store?"

Ages 9–12

Rikki Tikki Tavi
(1997) by Rudyard Kipling, New York: Candlewick Press

Highlight how "Rikki Tikki" is a rhyme. Challenge students to brainstorm a long list of words that rhyme with Rikki. Then, for each new character or location that is encountered in the story, have students generate a rhyme. For example:

> "Well, now we have Nag the cobra who has entered the story. Let's think of all the words we know that rhyme with Nag." *[Give students time to generate responses. List the words where all can see.]* "That's great! We thought of 13 words that rhyme with Nag's name. Let's continue with the story."

Phoneme Awareness

Ages 3–8

Sheep in a Shop

(1991) by Nancy Shaw, New York: Houghton Mifflin

This book is filled with phrases that contain matching initial sounds. For example, *hip/hooray, sheep/shop, rackets/rockets, buy/beach/ball, ribbon/rack, hop/home.* In addition, there is a rhyme on every page. Call children's attention to these matching initial sounds (i.e., alliteration) and rhymes. Challenge children to add words to each set of words that have matching initial sounds. For example:

> "Listen: *'Five sheep shop for a big, big day.'* Which 2 words in that sentence start with the *'sh'* sound?" *[Give children time to generate a response.]* "That's right, *sheep* and *shop*. They both have *'sh'* for their first sound. Let's think of 3 more words that start with *'sh.'"* *[Give children time to generate responses.]* "Great! We thought of *ship, shadow,* and *shoe*. We could say *'Five sheep shop for a ship, a shadow, and a shoe.'"*

To move to the phoneme manipulation level, challenge children to swap the initial sound in the alliterative word sets for a new sound to create a funny sentence. For example:

> "Listen: *'Sheep find rackets. Sheep find rockets.'* Which 2 words in those sentences start with the *'r'* sound?" *[Give children time to generate a response.]* "That's right, *rackets* and *rockets*. Now let's change the *'r'* sound to a *'p'* sound. What words do we get?" *[Give children time to generate responses.]* "That's right, *packets* and *pockets*. So it would be *'Sheep find packets. Sheep find pockets.'"*

Ages 9–12

Caddie Woodlawn

(1990) by Carol Ryrie Brink, New York: Aladdin Library

Many characters are represented in this book. Challenge students to substitute the initial sound in a person's name with the initial sound in their own names. For example:

> "Listen to this name: 'Caddie.' Now if we switch the /k/ in 'Caddie' with the /s/ at the beginning of my name, we get Saddie. Now, Michael, switch the first sound in Jane's name with the first sound in your name and tell us the new name." *[Give the student time to generate a response.]* "That's right. Mane is the new name. Nice work!"

To switch to a phoneme reversal task, have students reverse the phonemes in the different animals, foods, or locations that are in the story. For example:

> "Now Caddie is playing in the attic. Let's say the sounds in the word *attic* backwards together." *[Pronounce /kɪtæ/; encourage all students to respond.]*

References

Adams, M. (1990). *Beginning to read: Thinking and learning about print.* Cambridge, MA: MIT Press.

American Speech-Language-Hearing Association. (2001). *Scope of practice in speech-language pathology.* Rockville, MD: Author.

Blachman, B. (1989). Phonological awareness and word recognition: Assessment and intervention. In A. Kamhi and H. Catts (Eds.), *Reading disabilities: A developmental language perspective* (pp. 133–158). Boston: College Hill Press.

Blachman, B. (1991). Early intervention for children's reading problems: Clinical applications of the research in phonological awareness. *Topics in Language Disorders, 12(1),* 51–65.

Blachman, B. (Ed.). (1994). Early literacy acquisition: The role of phonological awareness. In G. Wallach and K. Butler (Eds.), *Language learning disabilities in school-age children and adolescents* (pp. 253–274). New York: Macmillan.

Bradley, L., & Bryant, P. E. (1983). Categorizing sounds and learning to read. *Nature, 301,* 419–421.

Bradley, L., & Bryant, P. E. (1985). *Rhyme and reason in reading and spelling.* Ann Arbor: University of Michigan Press.

Calfee, R. C. (1977). Assessment of independent reading skills: Basic research and practical applications. In A. S. Reber and D. L. Scarborough (Eds.), *Toward a psychology of reading* (pp. 289–323). New York: Erlbaum.

Catts, H. (1991). Facilitating phonological awareness: Role of speech-language pathologists. *Language, Speech, and Hearing Services in Schools, 22,* 196–203.

Catts, H. (2000, April). *Phonology, language, and reading: Implications for intervention.* Workshop presented for Dean Medical Center, Madison, WI.

Catts, H., Fey, M., Zhang, X., & Tomblin, B. (1999). Language basis of reading and reading disabilities: Evidence from a longitudinal investigation. *Journal of Scientific Studies of Reading, 3,* 331–362.

Catts, H., Fey, M., Zhang, X., & Tomblin, B. (2001). Estimating the risk of future reading difficulties in kindergarten children: A research-based model and its clinical implementation. *Language, Speech, and Hearing Services in Schools, 32,* 38–50.

Catts, H., & Kamhi, A. (1999). Causes of reading disabilities. In H. Catts and A. Kamhi (Eds.), *Language and reading disabilities* (pp. 95–127). Boston: Allyn and Bacon.

Content, A., Morais, J., Alegria, J., & Bertelson, P. (1982). Accelerating the development of phonetic segmentation skills in kindergartners. *Cahiers de Psychologie Cognitive, 2,* 259–269.

Ehri, L. (2000). Learning to read and learning to spell: Two sides of a coin. *Topics in Language Disorders, 20*(3), 19–36.

Feuerstein, R. (1980). *Instrumental enrichment.* Chicago: Scott Foresman.

Fey, M. (1999, Winter). Speech-language pathology and the early identification and prevention of reading disabilities. *Perspectives, 25,* 3–17.

Fey, M., Long, S., & Finestack, L. (2003). Ten principles of grammar facilitation for children with specific language impairments. *American Journal of Speech-Language Pathology, 12,* 3–15.

Gillon, G. (2000). The efficacy of phonological awareness intervention for children with spoken language impairment. *Language, Speech, and Hearing Services in Schools, 31,* 126–141.

Goldsworthy, C. (1998). *Sourcebook of phonological awareness activities.* San Diego, CA: Singular.

Gombert, J. (1992). *Metalinguistic development.* Chicago: University of Chicago Press.

Goswami, U., & Bryant, P. (1990). *Phonological skills and learning to read.* Hillsdale, NJ: Erlbaum.

Hall, S., & Moats, L. (1999). *Straight talk about reading.* Chicago: Contemporary Books.

Hodson, B. W. (2000, March). *Enhancing phonological and metaphonological skills.* Paper presented at the annual convention of the Wisconsin Speech-Language-Pathology and Audiology Association. Madison, WI.

Hodson, B. W., & Paden, E. P. (1991). *Targeting intelligible speech: A phonological approach to remediation.* Austin, TX: Pro-Ed.

Hoffman, P., & Norris, J. (1989). On the nature of phonological development: Evidence from normal children's spelling errors. *Journal of Speech and Hearing Research, 32,* 787–794.

Hubbard, C., & Mahanna-Boden, S. (2000, February). *Phonological awareness: Assessment and training activities.* Presentation at the annual convention of the Kentucky Speech-Language-Hearing Association, Louisville, KY.

Kamhi, A., & Catts, H. (1991). *Reading disabilities: A development language perspective.* Boston: Allyn and Bacon.

Leonard, L. (1991). Specific language impairment as a clinical category. *Language, Speech, and Hearing Services in Schools, 22,* 66–68.

Lewis, B., & Freebairn, L. (1992). Residual effects of preschool phonology disorders in grade school, adolescence, and adulthood. *Journal of Speech and Hearing Research, 35,* 819–831.

Lundberg, I., Frost, J., & Peterson, O. P. (1988). Effects of an extensive program for stimulating phonological awareness in preschool children. *Reading Research Quarterly, 23,* 263–284.

Martin, M., & Byrne, B. (2002). Teaching children to recognize rhyme does not directly promote phonemic awareness. *British Journal of Education Psychology, 72,* 561–572.

Masterson, J., and Crede, L.A. (1999). Learning to spell: Implications for assessment and intervention. *Language, Speech, and Hearing Services in Schools, 30,* 243–254.

Moats, L. (1995). *Spelling development, disability, and instruction.* New York: York Press.

Montgomery, J. (2001, April). *Literacy support for students with communication disabilities.* Paper resented at the annual convention of the Indiana Speech-Language-Hearing Association, Indianapolis, IN.

Muter, V., Hulme, C., Snowling, M., & Taylor, S. (1998). Segmentation, not rhyming, predicts early progress in learning to read. *Journal of Experimental Child Psychology, 71,* 3–27.

National Reading Panel. (2000). *Teaching children to read: An evidence-based assessment of the scientific research literature on reading and its implication for reading instruction.* Washington, DC: Department of Health and Human Services.

Nicolosi, L., Harryman, E., & Kresheck, J. (1996). *Terminology of communication disorders* (4th ed.). Baltimore: Williams and Wilkins.

Norris, J., & Hoffman, P. (1993). *Whole language intervention for school-age children.* San Diego, CA: Singular.

Northrup, P. S. (2002). *The literacy link.* Eau Claire, WI: Thinking Publications.

O'Connor, R. E., Jenkins, J. R., Leicester, N., & Slocum, T. A. (1993). Teaching phonological awareness to young children with learning disabilities. *Exceptional Children, 59,* 532–546.

O'Keefe, C. (2000, October). *Phonological awareness and the role of the speech-language pathologist in emergent literacy. Paper presented at the fall conference of the* Wisconsin Speech-Language Pathology and Audiology Association, Stevens Point, WI.

Perfetti, C. (1995). Cognitive research can inform reading education. *Journal of Research in Reading, 18*(2), 106–115.

Pring, L., & Snowling, M. (1986). Developmental changes in word recognition: An information processing account. *Journal of Experimental Psychology, 38A,* 395–418

Robertson, C., & Salter, W. (1995). *The Phonological Awareness Profile.* East Moline, IL: LinguiSystems.

Scarborough, H. (2001). Connecting early language and literacy to later reading (dis)abilities: Evidence, theory, and practice. In S. Neuman and D. Dickinson (Eds.), *Handbook of early literacy research* (pp. 97–110), New York: Guilford Press.

Silliman, E., & Wilkinson, L. C. (1994). Discourse scaffolds for classroom intervention. In G. Wallach and K. Butler (Eds.), *Language learning disabilities in school-age children and adolescents* (pp. 27–52). New York: Merrill.

Snow, C., Burns, M., & Griffin, P. (Eds.). (1998). *Preventing reading difficulty in young children.* Washington DC: National Academy Press.

Stackhouse, J. (1997). Barriers to literacy development in two cases of developmental verbal dyspraxia. *Cognitive Neuropsychology, 9,* 273–299.

Stanovich, K. E. (1988). *Children's reading and the development of phonological awareness.* Detroit, MI: Wayne State University Press.

Swank, L. (1997, November). Paper presented at the annual convention of the American Speech-Language-Hearing Association, Boston, MA.

Swank, L., & Catts, H. (1994). Phonological awareness and written word decoding. *Language, Speech, and Hearing Services in Schools, 25*(1), 9–14.

Torgesen, J. (1999). Assessment and instruction for phonemic awareness and word recognition skills. In H. Catts and A. Kamhi (Eds.), *Language and reading disabilities* (pp. 128–153). Neeham Heights, MA: Allyn and Bacon.

Torgesen, J., Wagner, R., & Rashotte, C. (1994). Longitudinal studies of phonological processing and reading. *Journal of Learning Disabilities, 27,* 776–786.

Treiman, R., & Baron, J. (1981). Segmental analysis ability: Development and relation to reading ability. In G. MacKinnon and T. Waller (Eds.), *Reading research: Advances in theory and practice* (pp. 159–198). New York: Academic Press.

Treiman, R., Zukowski, A., & Richmond-Welty, E. (1995). What happened to the "n" in *sink?* Children's spellings of final consonant clusters. *Cognition, 55,* 1–38.

van Kleeck, A. (1998). Preliteracy domains and stages: Laying the foundation for beginning reading. *Journal of Children's Communication Development, 20*(1), 33–51.

van Kleeck, A., Gillam, R., & McFadden, T. (1998). A study of classroom-based phonological awareness training for preschoolers with speech and/or language disorders. *American Journal of Speech-Language Pathology, 7*(3), 65–76.

Walsh, S. J. (2002). *Phonological awareness success: A step-by-step activity guide.* Eau Claire, WI: Thinking Publications.

Warrick, N., Rubin, H., & Rowe-Walsh, S. (1993). Phoneme awareness in language delayed children: Comparative studies and intervention. *Annals of Dyslexia, 43,* 153–173.

Watson, L., Layton, T., Pierce, P., & Abraham, L. (1994). Enhancing emerging literacy in a language preschool. *Language, Speech, and Hearing Services in Schools, 25,* 136–145.

Windsor, J., and Hwang, M. (1999). Derivational suffix productivity for students with and without language-learning disabilities. *Journal of Speech, Language, and Hearing Research, 42,* 220–230.